A Patient's Guide

Hope For Cancer Patients

Suffering with Chemotherapy Induced Peripheral Neuropathy

(CIPN)

Dr. Bao Thai, DC

Copyright © 2017 Bao Thai

All rights reserved.

ISBN-10: 1976140919

ISBN-13: 978-1976140914

Dedication

I wanted to sincerely thank everyone that has made this possible, especially my staff and my family. Without all of your support, my vision would never come true.

To my staff at Advanced Nerve and Laser: You are the best. You continue to strive and maintain a standard that is continuing to change people's lives! My vision of healing the world of nerve damage would not be possible without you.

To my parents Son and Du Thai. Since a child you have continued to help teach me what is important in life. You have given me the opportunity through your hard work and dedication to your family. I am able to do what I do today because of you.

To Suzanne and Connor, you are the reason why I work so hard. Suzanne, since the day we met, you have continued to push and support me. You have helped me become the man I am today. Every day we are together feels like the first time we met. There is no better person I could imagine life with than you!

Table of Contents

Section 1 8

   The Cell Cycle and Cancer 9

   How Does Chemo Treat Cancer? 14

   Why Do Chemotherapies Cause Peripheral Neuropathy? 16

   Which Chemotherapies Cause Peripheral Neuropathy? 21

      Bortezomib 23

      Carboplatin 24

      Cisplatin 26

      Cytarabine 28

      Docetaxel 29

      Oxaliplatin 30

      Paclitaxel 32

      Procarbazine 34

      Vinblastine 35

      Vincristine 35

   Dull the Symptoms: The Conventional Treatment 38

Why it is Important to Treat Chemotherapy-induced Neuropathy .38

Conventional Treatment Options.......40

Lyrica 43

Cymbalta 44

Neurontin 45

Conventional Treatment: Conclusion.46

The Outliers: Children who Recover from Chemo Induced Peripheral Neuropathy 48

Section 2 51

Start Today: How to Begin Treating Your Peripheral Neuropathy 51

Foods to Avoid 52

Foods to Eat 53

Supplementation................................54

Increase Blood Flow to your Nerves ..54

Simple Hand Exercises........................55

Simple Lower Extremity Exercises......55

Heal the Nerve: Continued Treatment ..58

What Further Treatment Looks Like ..58

Kill the Cancer, Not your Nerves: How to Limit Nerve Damage while Receiving Chemo Treatments 62

Why Treating Neuropathy *During* Chemotherapy is Different.................63

Section 3 66

What Hope Looks Like: Stories from People Who Fought Both Cancer and Neuropathy—and Won! 66

    Gerry S...66

    Illiana A...67

    Angelique R. 68

    Shaunte K. 69

    Bob M..70

From Hope to Freedom: Are you Ready for One More Battle?.............................71

Section 1

Cancer has changed your life. You fought back with chemotherapy. Sadly, the medicine that kills one condition has also created another: peripheral neuropathy. Peripheral neuropathy is an epidemic. It is a condition where your nerves are destroyed. In this case, it is because of chemotherapy. Symptoms can include (usually in the hands or feet):

- Burning
- Prickling pain
- Stabbing pain
- Tingling
- Numbness
- Weakness
- Inability to your digits
- Ataxia (difficulty walking)
- Painful sensitivity to heat or coldness
- Sensitivity to touch

In order to begin the journey of repairing your peripheral nervous system, you need to understand the cell cycle, cancer, and how chemotherapy works.

The goal of this book is for you to gain the knowledge that peripheral neuropathy can be reversed and that the results can be sustained! I understand that your doctors may have told you that there is nothing that can be done. I can tell you that is not true! We have helped and are helping patients just like you beat neuropathy every day. It is possible; you just have to make up your mind that you are going to do whatever it takes to beat the neuropathy as you did to beat cancer.

The Cell Cycle and Cancer

There are approximately 200 different types of tissue cells in your body. Cells like muscle cells, red blood cells, white blood cells, and nerve cells are the building blocks of your body.

The lifespan of a cell is called the cell cycle. Each cell goes through two main phases: interphase and mitosis. The interphase is the longest phase and is predominately spent growing the cell to a mature size and preparing for mitosis. Mitosis is the short phase the cell enters into at the end of its life to duplicate itself.

I promise I won't make you learn more than you need to. But in order to understand how chemotherapy has caused nerve damage, I have to touch on a few basics.

The Healthy Cell Cycle

Here is a list of the cell cycle phases and what happens with each phase:

- **G0** – This is the resting phase. The cell is performing its primary function and is not actively working towards cell division. Sometimes cells enter this phase through a process called contact inhibition. This means the cell recognizes that there are a sufficient number of other similar cells in the area and therefore cell division is not needed. Nerve cells remain in G0 indefinitely. Skin cells, on the other hand, never enter this phase.
- **G1** – The following three stages are all called the *interphase*. This is the process that allows the cell to gain the resources it needs to split into two daughter cells. G1 (otherwise known as "gap 1") causes the cell to increase in size and gather the necessary proteins it will need for the split.
- **S** – This is the synthesis phase. The cell is now actively duplicating its stored

DNA. Once this phase has completed, the cell will contain 46 *pairs* of chromosomes.
- **G2** – During this second gap phase, the cell grows even larger to support its future split while also beginning to develop the "tools" necessary (microtubules) to separate the chromosomes during the final division phase.
- **M** – The mitosis phase is comparatively short. Essentially, the nucleus wall—the envelope containing the duplicated chromosomes—disintegrates. Then the chromosomes organize themselves into a line in the middle of the cell. Microtubules form on the opposite poles of the cell and then reach out and pull the duplicated chromosomes apart—creating two separate copies. Finally, the cell walls collapse around the two distinct DNA strands and finally, two daughter cells are formed.

Here's the best part: if at any point during this process the cell realizes that it's damaged, it will prevent itself from completing mitosis. The cell will either permanently enter the G0 resting phase, or it will destroy itself through a process called apoptosis.

Here's the main takeaway: Each cell goes through stages while replicating itself. Once completed, the cell has become two exact copies called daughter cells. If the cell is damaged it will destroy itself to prevent damaged copies from being made.

What you'll see in a moment is that cancer doesn't follow the same rules.

The Cancerous Cell Cycle

Among other things, cancer cells have a "broken" cell cycle. Cancer forms when the cellular DNA has mutated in a way that the cell's natural safety features no longer work as intended.

First, cancer cells enter into mitosis faster, so they duplicate themselves more quickly. The cell cycle is shortened and they do not "rest."

Second, they no longer respond to contact inhibition. That means they'll continue to grow no matter how dense the surrounding tissue is.

These clumps of cancer cells are called neoplasms or tumors.

Third, they are invasive. Invasive growth causes the cancer cells to invade and destroy other tissue types surrounding the tumor.

Finally, the checkpoints that exist in the healthy cell cycle do not exist; therefore the cell does not destroy itself once it realizes that the DNA has been damaged.

There is a possibility that the mutations will continue to develop. This is how one cancer can grow and spread into another cancer.

Main Takeaways: Cancer cells have a broken cell cycle. They have mutated DNA that allows them to continue to replicate even though they no longer function as they ought. They are invasive and intrude into surrounding healthy tissue.

How Does Chemo Treat Cancer?

Chemotherapy is the use of medication to kill cancer cells. Obviously, if the substance indiscriminately killed cells you wouldn't call that medication; it would be a poison. Therefore, scientists have found ways to target certain cells for death and not others.

Chemotherapies work by interrupting the cell cycle. There are different types of chemotherapies and they act on different mechanisms, but what they have in common is that they prevent the cancer cells from growing through mitosis.

Most frequently, the drugs will either prevent mitosis or they will inhibit the copying of the DNA during the S phase of the cell cycle.

Unfortunately, there is no common way to target *only* cancer cells, so these drugs also attack healthy cells that are also in the targeted cell cycle phase.

Hair, intestine, and mouth cells are constantly replicating, and therefore chemotherapy patients have side effects of hair loss, nausea, and mouth sores. Those cells were killed at the same time they were killing the cancer cells.

Main Takeaway: Chemotherapies are lifesaving, cancer-killing drugs that function by interrupting the cell cycle. Because of the foreign attributes of cancer, those cells are damaged at a higher rate than healthy cells, but there are still damaging side-effects.

Why Do Chemotherapies Cause Peripheral Neuropathy?

As you already know, hair-loss and nausea are not the only side-effects of chemotherapy. These drugs also damage the peripheral nervous system.

A Brief Overview of the Nervous System

The nervous system is responsible for sending and receiving signals throughout the body. It is the system that responsible for purposeful movement, like closing your hand into a fist, or unconscious movements like breathing or stomach function. It is divided into two categories: the Central Nervous System and the Peripheral Nervous System.

The Central Nervous System is the brain, brain stem, and spinal cord. The Peripheral Nervous System connects to the central nervous system at the spine and reaches into your peripheries, like your hands and feet.

Nerve cells, or neurons, resemble a root ball with extended roots hanging off of them. The soma is the large portion that encloses the nucleus and the axon is a large branch that extends out into other tissue, sending and receiving electrical signals. The axon is insulated by a myelin sheath that ensures the signal is quickly relayed to the brain and it prevents signal distortion.

Unlike other cells, once a nerve cell has reached maturity, it becomes *post-mitotic*. This means it has completed its mitosis phase and will not enter it again. Because nerve cells do not go through mitosis, once a nerve cell is damaged, it is not replaced by a healthy cell.

Peripheral nerve cells come in two different varieties: sensory and motor. The whole point of sensory nerves is to communicate touch and feel between your external body and your brain. Motor nerves receive movement orders from your brain and cause the muscles to contract in the way your brain wanted.

Current research believes the area of your peripheral nervous system most affected by chemotherapy is the dorsal root ganglia. Let's take a minute to describe what that is and why it's important.

Now, imagine you are able to look down at yourself lying face-down on a table. You see your spine and the muscles of your back.

Hope for Cancer Patients

Inside your spine is the spinal cord. The spinal cord is made up of two different types of tissue: gray matter and white matter. If you were to hold a cross-section slice of your spinal cord, like a slice of bread, the center would look like a gray butterfly. That's the gray matter. The tops of the wings are towards your back and the bottom of the wings are pointing towards your front.

The white matter is made up of myelinated axons connecting the nerve bodies (gray matter) to the nerve branches outside of the spinal column. The roots coming out of the top of the butterfly-shaped gray matter is the dorsal root ganglia. These nerve bundles house a convergence of sensory and motor nerves.

If the dorsal root ganglia, this nerve bundle coming out of your spine, are damaged, it can affect both motor and sensory nerves in your extremities.

In this case, gravity is not on our side. You see your hands and feet are the farthest points away from the main part of your body. So circulation can be very hard for the body to do if you are on chemotherapy. The medication typically gets trapped at the extremities and causes the decline of the nerve.

Chemotherapy acts on weaknesses in the cell cycle defense. Your nerves are very exposed to the effects of chemotherapy because not only are they not protected by the blood–brain-barrier, but they require lots of blood to function correctly. This means that there is usually a relatively large amount of chemotherapy penetrating the nervous system.

Once inside the cell, chemotherapy can damage the nervous system in a variety of ways. In the next chapter, I'll discuss the most common chemotherapies and precisely how they damage the peripheral nervous system, but here are a few of the mechanisms:

- Chemotherapy destroys the myelin sheath surrounding the axon, causing disrupted signaling
- It can cause swelling in the dorsal root ganglia, affecting both your sensory and movement nerves
- It can prevent the mitochondria, "factories" providing power to each cell, from functioning or functioning well

Main Takeaways: A side-effect of their cancer-killing properties, chemotherapies also cause damage to nerve cells, some of which are found in the dorsal root ganglia.

Which Chemotherapies Cause Peripheral Neuropathy?

Each chemotherapy attacks cancer cells in different ways and at different times in the cell cycle, the way they cause peripheral neuropathy is varied as well. The following survey of peripheral neuropathy inducing chemotherapies is here as a reference work that you can use to better understand the possible damage caused by the chemotherapy your doctors prescribed you.

Before I continue, let me explain why I chose to use footnotes for this section. Due to the size and varied audience of this book, I thought it would be best to provide an overview of the different chemotherapies. Knowing the impact these drugs have had on your life, not only fighting cancer but also being the cause of neuropathy, I believed some of you might find it helpful to continue reading more on your particular drug.

The footnotes provided here were chosen because they covered that therapy in a way that I thought would be helpful to you. There is some overlap between the drugs, so I suggest you focus on the therapies that you have been

Hope for Cancer Patients

treated with and then proceed on to the next section of the book.

Remember, these additional resources were written by doctors and scientists for their fellow researchers, so they might not be easy to read.

You just need to grasp enough to understand how the treatment in the next section of the book can offer help.

Bortezomib[1]

Type of Treatment: Proteasome Inhibitor

Cancer Treated: Specific Blood cancers

Mechanism: The boron atom within the drug binds to a proteasome. Proteasomes are responsible for breaking down proteins. The proteins, in this case, are the ones that are responsible for causing apoptosis for cancer cells. If the proteins are broken down too quickly, then cancer does not destroy itself. With this treatment, the cell-death can now occur.

Cause for Peripheral Neuropathy: The mechanism for this side-effect is not yet known. One study reviewed the effects this drug had on animals after dosing. They noted damage to the myelin sheath and axonal degeneration to the animal neurons.[2,3] This

---

[1] Argyriou et al. Bortezomib-induced peripheral neuropathy in multiple myeloma: a comprehensive review of the literature. Blood. 2008;112:1593-1599. Blood. 2009;113(18):4478-4478. doi:10.1182/blood-2009-02-204206.

[2] Cavaletti G, Gilardini A, Canta A, et al. Bortezomib-induced peripheral neurotoxicity: A neurophysiological and pathological study in the rat. Experimental Neurology. 2007;204(1):317-325.

negatively impacted the transmission of electrical signals through the nerve cells.

Bortezomib is regularly connected to high complaints of peripheral neuropathy. Other than lowering, spacing out, or discontinuing the medication, no specific treatment has been found.

Carboplatin[4]

Type of Treatment: Platinum-based Antineoplastic (platin)

Cancer Treated: Varied, including ovarian, head, lung, neck, neuroblastoma, and brain.

Mechanism: Platin-family drugs prevent the duplication of DNA during the cell's synthesis (S) phase. If the DNA cannot be duplicated,

---

doi:10.1016/j.expneurol.2006.11.010.
[3] Meregalli C, Canta A, Carozzi VA, et al. Bortezomib-induced painful neuropathy in rats: A behavioral, neurophysiological and pathological study in rats. European Journal of Pain. 2010;14(4):343-350. doi:10.1016/j.ejpain.2009.07.001.
[4] Sousana Amptoulach and Nicolas Tsavaris, "Neurotoxicity Caused by the Treatment with Platinum Analogues," Chemotherapy Research and Practice, vol. 2011, Article ID 843019, 5 pages, 2011. doi:10.1155/2011/843019

then the cell cannot divide into two daughter cells.

Carboplatin is a second generation platin drug, deemed less toxic than its first generation cousin, cisplatin, but also less effective at treating certain cancers.

Cause for Peripheral Neuropathy: Up to 90% of patients receiving cisplatin experience some level of peripheral neuropathy. The higher the dose, the higher the likelihood of neuropathy and the level of neuropathy you will experience.

Patients receiving platin-family drugs and following conventional treatment plans will experience long-term neuropathy, and what little improvement patients describe, it is likely from sympathetic systems learning to adapt. For instance, some people experience difficulty in walking due to numbness. This can abate with increased adaptation in the legs and hips—they make up for where the feet are lacking.

Researchers show at least three ways that carboplatin causes peripheral neuropathy. First, the dorsal root ganglia are not protected by the blood–brain barrier as the brain is, so it is more susceptible to blood-borne toxins like chemotherapy. Second, the mechanism the cells use to fix NDNA (nuclear DNA) which is damaged by platin-family drugs, is less effective in nerve cells. Finally, there was a study that took cells from the dorsal root ganglia and a pheochromocytoma (a type of tumor). Both cell types had been treated with a platin-family drug. The study showed that the drug bound to the NDNA in DRG cells 10x more than the tumor cells. This could be because the cells are less-able to metabolize and remove platin drugs from within the cell.

Cisplatin

Type of Treatment: Platin

Cancer Treated: Varied, including ovarian, head, lung, neck, neuroblastoma, and brain.

Mechanism: Cisplatin, like other drugs in the platin-family, destroy cancer cells during any period in the cell cycle. They work by attacking the DNA of the cell, preventing it from duplicating.

Cause for Peripheral Neuropathy: Up to 90% of patients receiving cisplatin experience some level of peripheral neuropathy. The higher the dose, the higher the likelihood of neuropathy and the level of neuropathy you will experience.

Patients receiving platin-family drugs and following conventional treatment plans will experience long-term neuropathy, and what little improvement patients describe, it is likely from sympathetic systems learning to adapt.[5] For instance, some people experience difficulty in walking due to numbness. This can abate with increased adaptation in the legs and hips—they make up for where the feet are lacking.

Researchers show at least three ways that this drug causes peripheral neuropathy. First, the dorsal root ganglia are not protected by the blood–brain barrier as the brain is, so it is more susceptible to bloodborne toxins like chemotherapy. Second, the mechanism the cells use to fix NDNA (nuclear DNA) which is damaged by platin-family drugs, is less effective in nerve cells. Finally, there was a

---

[5] Siegal T, Haim N. Cisplatin-induced peripheral neuropathy. Frequent off-therapy deterioration, demyelinating syndromes, and muscle cramps. Cancer. 1990;66:1117-1123.

study that took cell from the dorsal root ganglia and a pheochromocytoma (a type of tumor). Both cell types had been treated with a platin-family drug. The study showed that the drug bound to the NDNA in DRG cells 10x more than the tumor cells. This could be because the cells are less-able to metabolize and remove platin drugs from within the cell.

Cytarabine

Type of Treatment: Antimetabolite and Nucleoside Analog families

Cancer Treated: A variety of leukemia and lymphomas

Mechanism: This drug blocks DNA polymerase which are enzymes that replicate a cell's DNA during the S phase of the cell cycle. When these enzymes are blocked, the cell is not able to divide.

Cause for Peripheral Neuropathy: This is a rare side effect of this chemotherapy. It was found in studies where researchers were using high doses of cytarabine.

Current studies are reviewing the direct effect this drug has on the nervous system. It seems that the drug causes damage to the myelin tissue which greatly affects nerve function.[6]

Docetaxel
Type of Treatment: Taxane

Cancer Treated: Breast, stomach, prostate, head and neck, non-small cell lunch cancer

Mechanism: The taxane-family of drugs affects the cells during the G2 and M phases of the cell-cycle. It works by creating microtubule dysfunction. The microtubules are responsible for pulling the centered pairs of DNA apart right before the cell splits into two daughter cells. When the microtubules are affected, they are no longer able to finish the DNA division. This causes the cell to die.

Cause for Peripheral Neuropathy: The taxane drugs invade the nerve cell mitochondria, damaging the axons, and in some cases, causing degradation to the nerve cells.[7]

---

[6] W J Baker, G L Royer Jr, and R B Weiss, "Cytarabine and neurologic toxicity." Journal of Clinical Oncology 9, no. 4 (April 1991) 679-93.
https://doi.org/10.1200/JCO.1991.9.4.679
[7] Tofthagen* C, McAllister RD, Visovsky C. Peripheral

Mitochondria are like power plants within the cell. Without functioning mitochondria, the nerve cell degrades.

Docetaxel induced peripheral neuropathy usually begins with "pins and needles," numbness, and loss of reflexes. These symptoms can progress to pain and ataxia, or problems with your gait while walking. Patients were most likely to encounter these symptoms at cumulative doses over 600mg.

Oxaliplatin
Type of Treatment: Platin

Cancer Treated: Varied, including ovarian, head, lung, neck, neuroblastoma, and brain.

Mechanism: Oxaliplatin, like other drugs in the platin-family, destroy cancer cells during any period in the cell cycle. They work by attacking the DNA of the cell, preventing it from duplicating.

Neuropathy Caused by Paclitaxel and Docetaxel: An Evaluation and Comparison of Symptoms. Journal of the advanced practitioner in oncology. 2013;4(4):204-215.

Cause for Peripheral Neuropathy: Up to 90% of patients receiving cisplatin experience some level of peripheral neuropathy. The higher the dose, the higher the likelihood of neuropathy and the level of neuropathy you will experience.

Patients receiving platin-family drugs and following conventional treatment plans will experience long-term neuropathy, and what little improvement patients describe, it is likely from sympathetic systems learning to adapt. For instance, some people experience difficulty in walking due to numbness. This can abate with increased adaptation in the legs and hips—they make up for where the feet are lacking.

Researchers show at least three ways that this drug causes peripheral neuropathy. First, the dorsal root ganglia are not protected by the blood–brain barrier as the brain is, so it is more susceptible to blood-borne toxins like chemotherapy. Second, the mechanism the cells use to fix NDNA (nuclear DNA) which is damaged by platin-family drugs, is less effective in nerve cells. Finally, there was a study that took cells from both the dorsal root ganglia and a pheochromocytoma (a type of tumor). Both cell types had been treated with a platin-family drug. The study showed that the drug bound to the NDNA in DRG cells 10x more than the tumor cells. This could be because the cells are less-able to metabolize and remove platin drugs from within the cell.

Ninety percent of patients receiving oxaliplatin are likely to experience temporary neuropathy that can pass within a few hours of the first infusion. They will experience tingling, numbness, and even some jaw tightening.

After four doses with a cumulative dose of over 540mg/m^2, the peripheral neuropathy patients experience is very similar to those receiving cisplatin.[8]

Paclitaxel
Type of Treatment: Taxane

Cancer Treated: Breast, stomach, prostate, head and neck, non-small cell lunch cancer

---

[8] V.A. Carozzi, et al., "Chemotherapy-induced peripheral neuropathy: What do we know about mechanisms?" Neurosci. Lett. (2014), http://dx.doi.org/10.1016/j.neulet.2s014.10.014

Mechanism: The taxane-family of drugs affects the cells during the G2 and M phases of the cell-cycle. It works by creating microtubule dysfunction. The microtubules are responsible for pulling the centered pairs of DNA apart right before the cell splits into two daughter cells. When the microtubules are affected, they are no longer able to finish the DNA division. This causes the cell to die.

Cause for Peripheral Neuropathy: The taxane drugs invade the nerve cell mitochondria, damaging the axons, and in some cases, causing degradation to the nerve cells.[9] Mitochondria are like power plants within the cell. Without functioning mitochondria, the nerve cell degrades.

Paclitaxel follows the "stocking and glove" pattern, which means the symptoms are focused on those areas covered by stockings and gloves. The symptoms are symmetrical, so both hands or feet will be affected. Burning, tingling, numbness, and loss of ability to feel vibration are frequently reported.[10]

---

[9] Tofthagen* C, McAllister RD, Visovsky C. Peripheral Neuropathy Caused by Paclitaxel and Docetaxel: An Evaluation and Comparison of Symptoms. Journal of the advanced practitioner in oncology. 2013;4(4):204-215.
[10] Eniu A. Weekly Administration of Docetaxel and

Procarbazine

Type of Treatment: Alkylating agent

Cancer Treated: Brain cancers, Hodgkin lymphomas

Mechanism: The mechanism by which procarbazine kills cancer is not fully understood. The evidence shows that it can prevent DNA synthesis.

Cause for Peripheral Neuropathy: This drug is frequently used along with other alkylating agents like vincristine.[11] When used by itself, procarbazine "less commonly" produces tingling and numbness in the hands and feet. Again, the mechanisms are not fully understood.

Paclitaxel in Metastatic or Advanced Breast Cancer. The Oncologist. 2005,10(9):665-685. doi:10.1634/theoncologist.10-9-665.

[11] Kim Y-J, Choe J, Park J-H, Hong Y-K. Efficacy of Procarbazine, Lomustine, and Vincristine Chemotherapy for Recurrent Primary Central Nervous System Lymphomas. Brain Tumor Research and Treatment. 2015;3(2):75-80. doi:10.14791/btrt.2015.3.2.75.

Vinblastine

Type of Treatment: Vinca-alkaloid

Cancer Treated: Hodgkin lymphoma

Mechanism: This drug binds to the tubulin protein which stops the cell from dividing the chromosomes during the M phase of the cell cycle. Once the cell separation is aborted at this phase, the cell dies.

Cause for Peripheral Neuropathy: Vinblastine, like vincristine, causes axonal swelling and nerve damage. It appears to directly affect the motor neurons. Patients have complained of difficulty walking and develop a foot-drop.[12]

Vincristine

Type of Treatment: Vinca-alkaloid

Cancer Treated: Most common chemotherapy used for pediatric cases. Various leukemias, Hodgkin's disease, and neuroblastoma, and small cell lung cancer.

---

[12] Suresh P, Kapoor R, Kapur BN. Severe neurotoxicity due to Vinblastine in Hodgkin lymphoma. South Asian Journal of Cancer. 2014;3(2):147-148. doi:10.4103/2278-330X.130492.

Mechanism: This drug binds to the tubulin protein which stops the cell from dividing the chromosomes during the M phase of the cell cycle. Once the cell separation is aborted at this phase, the cell dies.

Cause for Peripheral Neuropathy: This chemotherapy causes severe peripheral neuropathy.[13] What begins with tingling and burning in hands and feet later becomes painful cold sensitivity and loss of control of feet and hands.

Research shows that as vincristine interferes with the tubulin protein, it also causes axonal swelling and nerve tissue damage. While some research suggests that the peripheral neuropathy may improve after completing the chemotherapy, long term follow up with patients and a description of their continued symptoms has not been documented.

---

[13] Postma, T.J., Benard, B.A., Huijgens, P.C. et al., "Long term effects of vincristine on the peripheral nervous system." J Neuro-Oncol (1993) 15: 23. https://doi.org/10.1007/BF01050259

Dull the Symptoms: The Conventional Treatment

Why it is Important to Treat Chemotherapy-induced Neuropathy

It's one thing to read about numbness, tingling, burning, weakness, loss of balance and stability, loss of sense of vibration, and shooting pain on a symptom list. It's another thing to see how those symptoms can change the lives of real people.

When considered on their own, they may seem manageable, but when put in the context of a grandma, a teenager, a dad still trying to support his family, all of a sudden these symptoms can have effects that aren't readily apparent.

When was the last time you stepped on a nail and didn't know it? I've had patients do this multiple times. If you don't know you've hurt yourself, you won't take care of the wound. Infection can set it. You can re-injure yourself more easily as well.

How about you look at it from another perspective? How about the grandma that gets to do the one thing she wants to do: watch her

Hope for Cancer Patients

granddaughter during the day while her daughter works.

Then cancer.

That fight lasted years. She's in remission now, and she's hopeful that she can pick up her life where she last left it. But now that her feet have growing numbness and she's lost a great deal of strength, she can no longer carry her granddaughter up the many stairs in her house without fear of falling. The stairs are a necessary part of her house. As long as that fear is there, she can't risk being the only caretaker of her precious granddaughter.

She may have won the war, but cancer still managed to steal the one joy she had left.

That reads a lot different than "numbness" considered on its own, doesn't it?

Treating peripheral neuropathy isn't about managing symptoms, it's about putting your life back together.

So what are your options?

Conventional Treatment Options

The primary goal of chemotherapy is to cause cell death for cancer. That's its job. Sadly, over and over the research shows the number-one reason patients have to stop taking this life-saving therapy is that of debilitating peripheral neuropathy. Patients are able to work through the weakness, the hair loss, the nausea, but once the disabling numbness or the overwhelming pain of neuropathy sets in, it becomes unbearable.

In a very real way, peripheral neuropathy could be part of the way cancer kills its victims.

Doctors recognize this very real risk and have tried to meet this challenge as well as they can.

First, they have tried to find a method to prevent CIPN from developing in the first place. At this point, because of small study sizes and the fact that the mechanisms for chemotherapies are not all understood, there is no recommended method for preventing chemotherapy-induced peripheral neuropathy.[14]

---

[14] Hershman D. L., Lacchetti C., Dworkin R. H., Lavoie Smith E. M., Bleeker J., Cavaletti G., et al. . (2014). American Society of Clinical, Prevention and

Once patients begin experiencing peripheral neuropathy from chemotherapy, there is little hope it will lessen on its own. While some patients have found a partial resolution of peripheral neuropathy after receiving doses of oxaliplatin, others taking drugs like cisplatin, find that their symptoms continue to increase even after they've stopped getting chemotherapy.

So waiting around, hoping things get better is not an option.

Finally, doctors have tried treating CIPN, but sadly, they are limited to treating the symptoms, not the actual nerve and axonal damage that the chemotherapy caused.

The following are common medications and therapies for the conventional treatment of chemotherapy-induced peripheral neuropathy:

- NSAIDs like Ibuprofen can occasionally mask mild nerve pain

---

management of chemotherapy-induced peripheral neuropathy in survivors of adult cancers: American Society of Clinical Oncology clinical practice guideline. J. Clin. Oncol. 32, 1941–1967. 10.1200/JCO.2013.54.0914

- Antidepressant medications like amitriptyline or duloxetine hydrochloride
- Anticonvulsant medications like gabapentin
- Some epilepsy medications
- Steroids like Solu-Medrol or prednisone to reduce inflammation

When this doesn't work, and the pain is not sufficiently treated, doctors turn to narcotics to try to mask the pain. These medications are highly addictive and come with their own negative side-effects.

What you'll notice in the preceding list is that none of these meds are meant to heal your peripheral neuropathy. They take as a given that the nerve damage has happened, and the only hope they offer is to deaden what you are able to feel.

Aside from masking pain, these medications are going to continue to work as *they were originally designed*. Anti-depressant medications are going to affect your mood, and not necessarily in the same way they would for someone who actually needs the therapy.

And once you start down the road of narcotic pain medications, it's hard to find your way out.

Let's take a few moments and look at the most common medications prescribed to treat peripheral neuropathy, their effectiveness, and their common side effects.

Lyrica
Other Name: Pregabalin

Common Treatments: Traditional uses are to control seizures and treat fibromyalgia, also used for pain associated with nerve damage

General Information: Recent research has shown that many patients receiving Lyrica for peripheral neuropathy are not receiving the appropriate dose. Many patients needed a much higher dose to begin reporting a lower pain score.[15] This article does not discuss whether increased doses also created

---

[15] Serpell M, Latymer M, Almas M, Ortiz M, Parsons B, Prieto R. Neuropathic pain responds better to increased doses of pregabalin: an in-depth analysis of flexible-dose clinical trials. Journal of Pain Research. 2017;Volume 10:1769-1776. doi:10.2147/jpr.s129832.

increased side-effects. It should also be noted that the researchers were working for Pfizer, the pharmaceutical company.

Common Side Effects Include: Ataxia, tremors, tingling, constipation, drowsiness, weight gain, accidental injury.

Many of the side-effects of this drug are also the symptoms of peripheral neuropathy. It appears to be treating the painful symptoms of peripheral neuropathy by replacing them with the numbing symptoms.

Cymbalta
Other Name: Duloxetine

Common Treatments: Major Depressive Disorder (adults), general anxiety disorder, nerve pain, and fibromyalgia

General Information: Cymbalta is a serotonin and norepinephrine reuptake inhibitor. Researchers believe that by increasing the levels of serotonin and norepinephrine in the brain and nervous system, your body masks the pain signals your damaged nerves are sending. This isn't treating the nerves themselves, rather it is, in a sense, muting the signals those nerves are sending.

Common Side-Effects: Dizziness, drowsiness, headaches, sedation, fatigue, psychomotor agitation (less common), nausea

Neurontin
Other Name: Gabapentin

Common Treatments: Viral nerve pain, seizures, Restless Leg Syndrome

General Information: By binding to particular calcium channels in the nervous system, this medication attenuates peripheral nerve pain. Due to the increased push to prevent doctors from prescribing opioids for pain, they have begun prescribing drugs like Neurontin (gabapentin) more and more, even though the results don't always prove that it's effective.[16]

Common Side-Effects: Drowsiness, fatigue, ataxia, nystagmus (eye tremors), fever,

---

[16] Goodman CW, Brett AS. Gabapentin and Pregabalin for Pain — Is Increased Prescribing a Cause for Concern? *New England Journal of Medicine*. 2017;377(5):411-414. doi:10.1056/nejmp1704633.

peripheral swelling, tremors, suicidal thoughts (rarer)

Conventional Treatment: Conclusion

Over and over you read the side effects of these medications and one thing that they all have in common is that they share symptoms with peripheral neuropathy.

Even if you do find relief from your pain with these medications, it's important to note that they are only masking the pain and irritation signals your damaged nervous system is sending.

These drugs don't make you better.

You beat cancer. You are trying to beat peripheral neuropathy, and now you have to fight the side-effects of the meds that are trying to treat the side-effects of the meds that killed your cancer. Yes. It's that crazy.

It's not fair.

But you aren't alone.

It can feel like there's no hope.

But there is one group of patients who *do* seem to improve from chemotherapy-induced neuropathy.

Maybe there's hope after all…

The Outliers: Children who Recover from Chemo Induced Peripheral Neuropathy

There was a study done a few years back that looked at how quickly kids recovered from chemotherapy-induced peripheral neuropathy.[17] The article doesn't say anything about how they were treated for the symptoms, but as we already covered, if they received any treatment, it was just to mask the symptoms.

All of the children were exposed to vincristine, as it is the most effective drug to treat childhood cancers. It also happens to be one of the most toxic to your peripheral nervous system.

In fact, there are quite a few case studies where a child inadvertently had vincristine injected into the spinal column—in direct contact with the cerebrospinal fluid—and it in almost every case leads to a nervous system shutdown and death.[18]

---

[17] Gilchrist L. S., Tanner L. R., Ness K. K. (2017). Short-term recovery of chemotherapy-induced peripheral neuropathy after treatment for pediatric non-CNS cancer. Pediatr. Blood Cancer 64 180–187. 10.1002/pbc.26204

Hope for Cancer Patients

Now, here's what I found most interesting. The kids that had the lowest score on the peripheral neuropathy test were also the kids who had the most vincristine. They're also the kids that showed the most improvement 6 months after completing chemotherapy.

So either vincristine isn't as neurotoxic as everyone says it is, or there's another variable.

The kids that scored the best were the youngest kids. The older the kids were, the less they recovered (as a whole).

Now, the conclusion of this study essentially stated that more research needs to be completed before any final conclusions should be drawn.

But the fact that the youngest kids healed the most doesn't really surprise anyone. Even though we know that nerve cells don't replace themselves through mitosis, there is still a way for damaged nerves and axons to repair themselves, and it appears to be most active in kids.

---

[18] Shepherd DA, Steuber CP, Starling KA, Fernbach DJ. Accidental intrathecal administration of vincristine. Medical and Pediatric Oncology. 1978;5(1):85-88. doi:10.1002/mpo.2950050113.

I began reading everything I could on recovery from chemotherapy-induced peripheral neuropathy in children. If your body could repair itself at 5, maybe there was a way for it to repair itself at 50.

After thousands of patients and countless hours reading and studying, I've found at least part of the answer.

The secret is creating a process that would allow your body to have the resources as if you were a child. There are certain proteins that must be produced by the cell for the nerves to grow. Specifically, we are talking about GAP43. Once GAP43 is produced and you're able to produce an environment where the body is in a regenerative and reparative mode. The results are we get repair in the nerve.

Section 2

Start Today: How to Begin Treating Your Peripheral Neuropathy

You are now going to learn how to tell your body it needs to begin healing your damaged nerves, just like it would do automatically if you were a young child.

To begin healing, you need to find a way to reduce the inflammation in your body. The best way to do this is to begin eating anti-inflammatory foods.

Inflammation is part of your body's innate immune system. This is a process that begins whenever there has been cellular damage.

Remember the last time you were scratched? Your skin became raised around the area where it was cut, creating a large welt along the length damage The skin was warm to the touch and you may have seen additional swelling.

That's inflammation. While it may be uncomfortable, it's a useful tool your body uses to bring healing to damaged tissue. It does this by aiding apoptosis, flushing out damaged cellular material, and creating an environment for cell growth.

But when you have damage by chemotherapy, that inflammation can become chronic inflammation. Inflammation is supposed to bring about healing, but when it becomes chronic, it actually creates an environment that is killing cells and healing cells at the same time. It's a never-ending cycle.

The foods you eat can either exacerbate or reduce inflammation.

Foods to Avoid
You should avoid the following foods as much as you can. I know it can be hard to make some changes, but the goal is to create an environment inside your body that helps your nerves begin the healing process.

- Sugar
- Fried foods
- Artificial preservatives
- Refined flour
- Red meats

Hope for Cancer Patients

- Processed food

Let's make this easy: If it comes in a box, it's more than likely going to cause inflammation.

Foods to Eat

These foods work with your body to bring down the inflammation process that will help your body heal. By the way, I've listed the "fun" foods at the end.

- Green tea
- Broccoli
- Blueberries
- Wild Salmon
- Garlic
- Most fresh vegetables
- Black beans
- Oysters
- Yogurt
- Nuts
- Bone Broth
- Honey
- Dark chocolate

Basically, the opposite of what was true with inflammation is true with anti-inflammatory foods: the fresher, more natural a food is, the more likely it'll be working to help you heal your peripheral neuropathy.

Supplementation
Head to your local vitamin store and add the following supplements to your daily diet:

- Omega-3 fatty acids
- Alpha lipoic acid
- B-vitamins like L-Carnatine and Thiamine

Research has shown that these supplements will improve neurological function. Again, you want to give yourself every chance to succeed.

Increase Blood Flow to your Nerves
Now that you are creating the right environment for your nerves to heal, you need to make sure they are getting plenty of blood flow. Without blood, tissues atrophy and die—and that is exactly what you are trying to reverse.

The point of these exercises is not to make you break out in a sweat, but to make sure you have a full range of motion through the joints

Hope for Cancer Patients

closest to where the neuropathy has set in. This will ensure the affected digit or area has an increase in blood flow.

Simple Hand Exercises

1. Twiddle your thumbs—clasp your fingers together and circle your thumbs around each other. Then begin circling your other fingers around each other, one at a time.
2. Press your thumb and finger tip together in an "a-ok sign." Now slide your thumb down the extent of your finger. Now reverse and slide your finger down the extent of your thumb. Continue through all of your fingers.

Increase your grip strength by squeezing something with resistance for 10 seconds at a time as tightly as you can. You can start really light by rolling up a washcloth and using that as your resistance. Move your way up to something like a tennis ball.

Simple Lower Extremity Exercises

1. Sit in a chair and stretch out your foot in front of you. Now, imagine you are trying to swirl some water with your toes. Point your toes and rotate your foot around, first clockwise and then counterclockwise. Repeat with your other foot.
2. Now, with your feet flat on the floor, lift your toes up as high as they can go and then bring them down until they tap on the floor. You can do these seated or standing, feet together or apart. Consider changing it up every few days. The variation will cause you to use different stabilizer muscles.
3. Finally, do some useful movement like walking or stepping up and down stairs. Go slowly. You aren't going to worry about distance covered or speed, rather just focus on correct motion. Step heel-to-toe. Be deliberate and feel your foot roll on the ground.

These simple additions to your day will begin to create an environment where your nerves have the best chance at healing. Start slowly and work your way up.

As you work on functional movement like squeezing and walking, you'll also strengthen secondary systems that will also help you improve your capabilities.

Heal the Nerve: Continued Treatment

The last chapter hit on three main areas to begin helping your body regenerate your peripheral nerves. Those three areas are:

- Reducing inflammation
- Increasing blood flow
- Providing your body with the supplements and proteins you need to rebuild the nervous tissue

The patients that come see me work on those same things with some added tools.

What Further Treatment Looks Like

When someone calls my office wanting help with neuropathy, I always call them at home first. I don't want to waste their time driving to my office if their situation is one that I can't help.

During our conversation, I'll ask you about what cancer you were diagnosed with and what chemotherapies your doctor used to treat you.

Then we'll discuss your current symptoms. I'll want to know how your current pain or numbness also impacts your daily activities.

If your situation is one that I think I can help with, we'll have you come in for an in office consultation.

The first appointment will last approximately 90 minutes. I'll take a longer medical history and then see if I can identify the nerves that are damage. Once that is establish we will run through a process where we can see if your nerves will respond to my process.

If your peripheral nervous system's environment can be changed, you will see the results immediately. So I'll isolate a nerve and begin a small version of the treatment program you would begin if this works. This will involve laser therapy to initiate a change in the nerve and its environment, as well as other elements to wok on reducing inflammation.

Now it's up to you. If you feel an improvement, then it would seem that your neuropathy will respond to treatment. If you tell me that you don't feel any different, then I don't want to waste your time trying to treat nerves that won't respond.

If you tell me that you responded to the treatment, then I'll get you started on a tailored program that will look at what specific treatments are needed to treat your exact symptoms, particular supplements to provide your body the building blocks for neurological regeneration, and some diet adjustments to reduce inflammation.

You'll also take some medical equipment home with you that will help your body improve blood flow and help control the pain. You'll come see me 1-2 times a week, but you'll be working on healing every day.

Here's what I've seen after treating thousands of patients.

1. 50% of all the people that see me for an initial appointment respond to the treatment and continue on (although the average is higher for chemotherapy patients).
2. Approximately 93% of the people who continue on, leave with either no symptoms or drastic improvement. Chemotherapy patients usually respond better than the average, because the cause of the nerve damage

(chemo) has stopped, unlike other patients with different diseases.
3. Most patients complete treatment in 8 weeks, but some continue treatment and finish in 16 weeks. This is not something that requires perpetual treatment. You've completed chemotherapy; let's help your body heal from the damage.

I hope you are beginning to believe that the neuropathy you are experiencing doesn't have to be permanent. Your body was made to heal. Studies prove that the peripheral nervous system can regenerate in certain circumstances. The treatment described in this book teaches you how to create that perfect environment.

But what if you are still undergoing chemotherapy? What if the damage is ongoing for the foreseeable future? That's what the next chapter is all about.

Kill the Cancer, Not your Nerves: How to Limit Nerve Damage while Receiving Chemo Treatments

This chapter could be the most important thing I've ever written. I'm not trying to be dramatic. In fact, I can even back it up with research.

The number one reason oncologists have to back down on chemotherapy doses or change chemotherapies is peripheral neuropathy.

Let me state that another way.

The number one reason doctors have to stop aggressively killing cancer is peripheral neuropathy.

That's how incredibly life-changing peripheral neuropathy can be. Patients will choose to not fight cancer as hard as their doctor thinks they should because it hurts too much, or because they are becoming disabled by the chemo.

I want you to fight cancer as hard as you can. I want you to win and then go live your life with renewed vigor and purpose, knowing you've fought one of the hardest enemies we face.

Hope for Cancer Patients

So let's take a few minutes and talk about what it will take to keep peripheral neuropathy from taking you out of the fight.

Why Treating Neuropathy *During* Chemotherapy is Different

When I treat someone post-chemotherapy, I have a pretty good idea what kind of nerve damage has been done, and that means I have an idea of how much work it will take to bring some healing.

When you are getting chemotherapy, the drug is actively causing nerve damage. Patients at this stage actually have a lot more in common with diabetes patients—their disease is actively causing nerve damage too.

During this phase, our goal is to limit the amount of peripheral nerve damage you experience instead of trying to heal the nerves and reverse the damage.

I believe in being straightforward with my patients. While I have seen patients go through concurrent therapy with me and chemo, and never experience peripheral neuropathy, it's far more common to have a patient go through their chemo course with some peripheral nerve damage.

But where they *end* chemotherapy is much better than where most of my patients *start* with me after they've completed chemo.

Once you have stopped chemotherapy treatments, we can work together to reverse the nerve damage and heal your neuropathy symptoms.

So, let's assume you are taking chemotherapy right now. What should you do?

First, you need to set the right expectations. Your goal for your mental state is to keep it together to finish your chemotherapy. That's most important.

Cancer has and will change you. Very few people leave chemotherapy with no side-effects. Don't expect to be one of the outliers.

But that doesn't mean there's nothing you can or should do to fight those side effects. Let's make sure you are fighting as hard as you can on all fronts.

Second, you need to keep moving. Nerves need blood flow to live. As we've already covered in the exercise section of the book. Even though it'll be uncomfortable, painful, or just downright hard, you need to keep your limbs moving.

Finally, you need to take care of yourself. Get as much sleep as your body needs (hint, that's at least 8hrs a night). Take time to eat a healthy, low-inflammation diet. Consider asking friends or family to help you with cooking. If you call my office, I can send you my favorite healthy-nerve recipes.

This may seem simple enough, but trust me, if you turn these three things into habits each day, you can get through your chemotherapy treatment better than you expect.

If you want more advice, you can always give me a call. We can discuss your situation and see what other options might be available.

Section 3

What Hope Looks Like: Stories from People Who Fought Both Cancer and Neuropathy—and Won!

Gerry S.
I was diagnosed with Rectal Cancer in January 2014 and with Inflamed Nodes in my pelvic area in February 2016! Little did I know that this health journey over 2 ½ years would wind through 26 rounds of chemotherapy, 6 weeks of radiation, major surgery to my abdominal area, a wound that would not heal, a home health nurse coming to my house 3 times a week to help me navigate the changes going on with my body and bringing me to a mobility challenge that would stifle my independence, upset my daily living routine, cause me to fall repeatedly and have to change my very way of life!

I was introduced to Dr. Thai via Good Morning Texas when he and Dennis (his first patient to appear with him discussing Neuropathy) back in September 2015. By that time, I was

Hope for Cancer Patients

dragging my right leg, not working, driving what amounted to a 10-mile radius around my home and not feeling as if I was contributing much else.

Simple things like driving, cooking, cleaning, walking, sitting on a standard chair or toilet (or getting up from said chair or toilet), climbing stairs or kneeling – could not be done!

Today I am a new man! I can do all the things I want to do. I am having no problems at all with the neuropathy! I'm excited each day that I'm able to walk around without my "medical walking stick" (fancy name for a cane)!

I CANNOT thank Dr. Thai and his team at Advance Nerve and Laser enough for their professionalism, their energy, and efficiency in the office! Dr. Thai is doing a marvelous work indeed! He is restoring hope, independence and shining a light on unconventional methods of healing and restoration at a time when it is needed most!

Illiana A.

I had breast cancer. I developed neuropathy in my hands and feet after chemo therapy treatments. I had a mastectomy in October of 2015. I noticed numbness and tingling after chemo treatments. I was not even able to sleep through the night. The doctors did a lot of nerve studies and told me I had neuropathy. I didn't know what it was or how serious it was. They gave me medication to control it I told the doctors I wouldn't take any of the drugs without knowing what caused the symptoms. I started my investigation and research and discovered that there is no cure for neuropathy. I refused to be in a wheelchair. On Valentine's Day I turned the TV on and I watched Dr. Thai. I called immediately to see if I could get in. I am able to work for an hour at my desk doing paperwork without the chronic pain. My life has changed completely.

Angelique R.

I had stage 4 breast cancer. After chemo, I developed neuropathy. My nerves were damaged from the thighs down. I had shooting pains, I was in bed, and I was on all kinds of pain medications. The quality of life was bad and I had two small children. It was affecting my life. I saw Dr. Thai on Good Morning Texas. I told myself, "I have got to give this a go. What do I have to lose? I can't keep laying here the rest of my life." I'm feeling good. I work out; I try to work out every day. I'm running around with my kids. I'm involved with the school now. I'm not in bed. I'm off all the pills. No more pills. It's awesome!

Shaunte K.

I took a fall in January and I was walking around fine toward the end of my chemotherapy treatment. There were no treatments that were recommended by physicians. I went to a neurologist because there was no explanation as to why I suddenly had the challenges in walking and balance. You can imagine how concerning that was when he said I see nothing wrong. I am extremely independent and I was losing my independence and that was a struggle. Having to ask my husband and children to take me where I needed to go because I wasn't able to get in the car and drive was humiliating. I was at physical therapy and they were trying to change it up and see if maybe changing the program up could stimulate my body just a little more. I was riding the bike and I hear this guy in the background talking and he was saying, "My feet feel like lead." He then described everything he couldn't do anymore. I turned around and looked at the television and I said "Oh my gosh. Did I just script that? I mean what was going on?" Literally tears start running down my face. Today we have a family tracker on our phones. My husband is tracking me to see where I am. When modern medicine, even when conventional medicine is telling you that there is absolutely nothing wrong. I'm not really sure why you are experiencing what you are experiencing. Hearing him talk about there is still an option. You have no idea the feeling I felt.

Bob M.

I got neuropathy from chemotherapy. I came in with my feet with burning and numb. I had no feeling from the bottom of my feet to my toes. I also had pain in my legs as well as burning. After going through Dr. Thai's program I am happy to say I have no more neuropathy. My feet are good with problems. I am able to walk and do the things I wanted to do with out the fear of falling. I am so happy and grateful for Dr. Thai and his staff.

From Hope to Freedom: Are you Ready for One More Battle?

You need to be informed. You need to know why you are hurting. You need to think through the impact it is having on your life.

Like I've shown through stories of real cancer-survivors already, "numbness" doesn't begin to explain the impact peripheral neuropathy can have on your life.

By this point, you understand the basics of how cancer grows and the various mechanisms that chemotherapy uses to kill it.

You also know that the unintended result of this life-saving medication is nerve damage that can change your life.

You understand that diet, exercise and lifestyle changes can have a dramatic impact on your life, and help you regain some of what you've lost to nerve damage.

You might think that I spend most of my time with my patients performing procedures or teaching them about the mechanisms of disease.

You'd be wrong.

I spend most of my time helping my patients find hope.

After everything you've been through, it's easy to give up when one hurdle after another bars your way.

My desire is that I've helped you find hope now.

If peripheral neuropathy is destroying your life more than you can tolerate, if you are at the point where you see that your independence is going away, if you are ready to get your life back, my staff and I am here for you.

If you want to see more real success stories visit www.nerveandlaser.com.

It's time for you to start living again! My vision is to heal the world of nerve damage and it all starts with you. Reach out to me today so I can help give your life back!

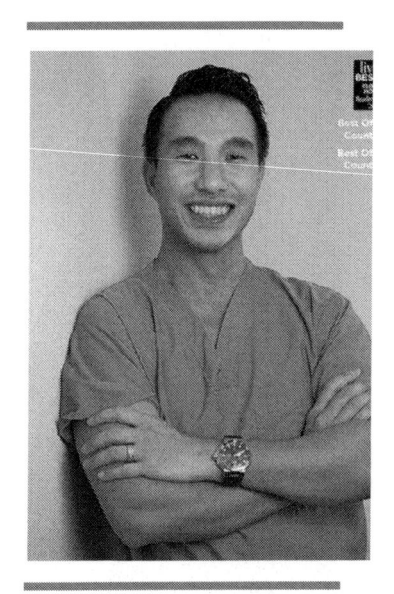

About the Author

Dr. Bao Thai, DC, is a #1 international best-selling author on the topic of nerve damage and has spent over 11 years in healthcare helping patients around the world. Dr. Thai has appeared on ABC, CBS, NBC, and FOX stations around the US and has been featured in magazines and newspapers. He has spoken at Harvard. He has won numerous awards for the best doctor such as:

- 2015 Best of Denton County
- 2016 Best of Denton County

- 2017 Best of Denton County
- 2016 Living Magazine
- 2017 Living Magazine
- 2017 Harvard Pain Innovations
- 2016 Super Doc
- 2017 Super Doc

Dr. Thai specializes in helping patients find solutions for their nerve problems when conventional treatments fail. He uses technology and proprietary system to help change his patient's lives. He is a devoted father and husband.

Dr. Thai is on a mission to end all nerve damage!